The Complete Diabetes Cookbook

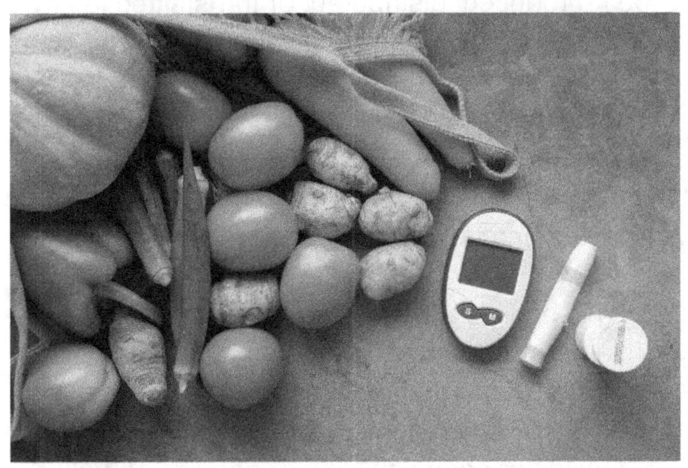

Healthy, Nutritious and Delicious Meals to Longevity and a Healthier you

Isaac Hendricks

Table of Contents

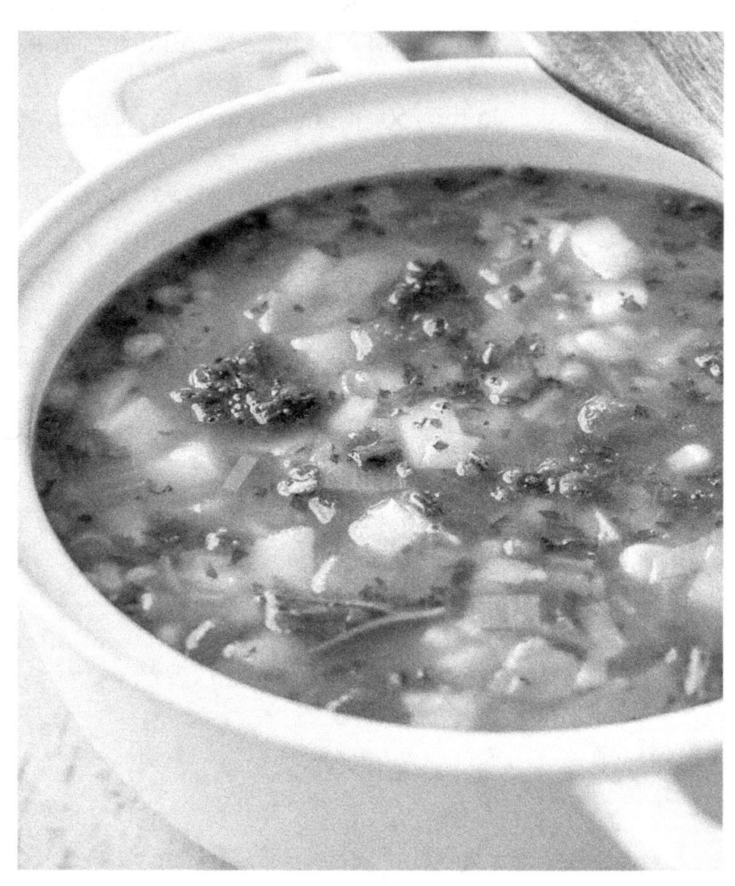

INTRODUCTION

Welcome to "The Complete Diabetes Cookbook," a culinary journey designed to empower individuals with diabetes to embrace a delicious and nutritious approach to everyday meals. Whether you're navigating the challenges of managing diabetes or seeking fresh inspiration for a health-conscious lifestyle, this cookbook is your trusted companion on the path to flavorful and mindful eating.

Living with diabetes involves making informed choices about food, and this cookbook is crafted to make those choices not only manageable but enjoyable. In this introductory section, let's explore the key components that set the tone for the rest of the book.

1. Understanding Diabetes:
Diabetes is a complex condition, and understanding its basics is crucial for effective management. We delve into the fundamentals, explaining the different types of diabetes, how the body processes insulin, and the impact of blood sugar levels on overall health. This knowledge lays the foundation for making informed choices in the kitchen.

2. Importance of Nutrition in Diabetes Management:
Nutrition plays a pivotal role in managing diabetes. In this section, we discuss the significance of a

well-balanced diet, focusing on the right mix of carbohydrates, proteins, fats, vitamins, and minerals. Discover how making thoughtful food choices can positively impact blood sugar levels and contribute to overall well-being.

3. **Tips for Cooking and Eating Mindfully:**
Mindful eating is a key component of diabetes management. Explore practical tips for cultivating mindfulness in the kitchen and at the table. From savoring each bite to understanding portion control, these insights will help you build a positive relationship with food while managing your diabetes effectively.

Embark on this culinary adventure with the confidence that comes from understanding the foundations of diabetes management and the role that nutrition plays in your journey. "The Complete Diabetes Cookbook" goes beyond being a collection of recipes; it's a comprehensive guide that empowers you to make informed and enjoyable choices in your daily culinary experiences. So, let's start cooking with a purpose — to nourish both body and soul.

CHAPTER ONE

Understanding Diabetes

Diabetes is a complex and chronic medical condition that occurs when the body struggles to regulate blood sugar, or glucose, effectively. To grasp the nuances of diabetes, it's essential to explore the types, causes, and mechanisms that underlie this condition.

1. Types of Diabetes:
- Type 1 Diabetes: This form of diabetes is characterised by the immune system mistakenly attacking and destroying insulin-producing beta cells in the pancreas. People with Type 1 diabetes require insulin injections to manage their blood sugar levels.

- Type 2 Diabetes: In this more common type, the body either doesn't produce enough insulin or becomes resistant to its effects. Lifestyle, genetics, and weight are frequently linked to Type 2 diabetes.

2. Insulin and Blood Sugar Regulation:
- Role of Insulin: Insulin is a hormone produced by the pancreas that facilitates the absorption of glucose into cells for energy.

In diabetes, this process is interrupted, resulting in high blood sugar levels.

- Blood Sugar Fluctuations: Maintaining blood sugar levels within a specific range is crucial for overall health. High blood sugar (hyperglycemia) and low blood sugar (hypoglycemia) can have immediate and long-term consequences.

3. Risk Factors and Causes:

- Genetic Factors: Family history can contribute to the risk of developing diabetes.

- Lifestyle Factors: Sedentary lifestyles, poor dietary choices, and obesity can increase the likelihood of Type 2 diabetes.

- Autoimmune Factors: Type 1 diabetes is often triggered by an autoimmune response.

4. Complications of Diabetes:

- Cardiovascular Issues: Diabetes increases the risk of heart disease and stroke.

- Neuropathy and Nerve Damage: Elevated blood sugar levels can lead to nerve damage, causing tingling or numbness.

- Kidney Problems: Diabetes is the major cause of renal failure.

- Eye Complications: Diabetes can contribute to vision problems and blindness.

5. Management and Treatment:
- Lifestyle Modifications: Healthy eating, regular physical activity, and weight management play pivotal roles in diabetes management.

- Medications: Insulin and various oral medications may be prescribed to control blood sugar levels.

- Monitoring: Regular monitoring of blood sugar levels is essential for adjusting treatment plans.

Understanding diabetes is the first step towards effective management. With this knowledge, individuals can make informed lifestyle choices, engage in proactive healthcare, and work towards achieving a balanced and fulfilling life despite the challenges posed by this condition. Consult a healthcare professional for personalized advice and treatment.

Importance of Nutrition in Diabetes Management

Nutrition is a cornerstone in the effective management of diabetes, playing a crucial role in controlling blood sugar levels, preventing complications, and promoting overall well-being. Here's an exploration of the key aspects highlighting the importance of nutrition in diabetes management:

1. Balancing Macronutrients:

- carbs: Understanding the effects of carbs on blood sugar is critical. Choosing complex carbohydrates with a low glycemic index helps regulate blood sugar levels more steadily.

- Proteins: Including lean proteins supports satiety and helps stabilise blood sugar levels.

- Fats: Opting for healthy fats, such as those found in avocados and nuts, contributes to heart health and can assist in managing insulin resistance.

2. Portion Control:

- Moderation in portion sizes is vital for individuals with diabetes. It helps prevent spikes in blood sugar levels and assists in maintaining a healthy weight.

3. Meal Timing:

- Distributing meals evenly throughout the day helps prevent extreme fluctuations in blood sugar. Consistent meal timing, including healthy snacks, can support better glycemic control.

4. Fibre-Rich Diet:

- High-fibre foods, such as whole grains, fruits, and vegetables, have numerous benefits for individuals with diabetes. Fibre aids in digestion, helps control blood sugar levels, and contributes to a feeling of fullness.

5. Monitoring Glycemic Index:

- Understanding the glycemic index of foods assists in making informed choices. Foods with a lower glycemic index are digested more slowly, causing a gradual rise in blood sugar levels.

6. Hydration:

- Staying well-hydrated is crucial for everyone, but particularly for individuals with diabetes. Water helps regulate blood sugar levels, supports kidney function, and aids in digestion.

7. Individualised Approach:

- Every person with diabetes is unique, and there is no one-size-fits-all approach to nutrition. Tailoring dietary choices to individual needs, preferences, and tolerances is essential for effective management.

8. Weight Management:

- Maintaining a healthy weight is beneficial in diabetes management. Nutrition plays a central role in achieving and sustaining weight goals, contributing to better blood sugar control.

9. Collaboration with Healthcare Professionals:

- Working closely with healthcare providers, including dietitians and nutritionists, ensures personalised guidance. These professionals can help create a balanced and sustainable meal plan that aligns with individual health goals.

In summary, the importance of nutrition in diabetes management cannot be overstated. It serves as a powerful tool for individuals to take control of their health, optimise blood sugar levels, and reduce the risk of complications associated with diabetes. Adopting a well-balanced and mindful approach to nutrition is a cornerstone in the journey toward a healthier and more fulfilling life with diabetes.

Tips for Cooking and Eating Mindfully

Mindful cooking and eating can significantly enhance the experience of managing diabetes by fostering a deeper connection with food and promoting healthier choices. Here are practical tips to cultivate mindfulness in the kitchen and at the dining table:

1. Engage Your Senses:
- Begin by appreciating the colours, textures, and aromas of the ingredients. Engaging your senses enhances the overall cooking and dining experience.

2. Focus on the Present Moment:
- When cooking, concentrate on each task at hand. Avoid multitasking to fully immerse yourself in the process, promoting a sense of calm and enjoyment.

3. Portion Awareness:
- Be mindful of portion sizes, using smaller plates if needed. This practice helps prevent overeating and supports better blood sugar control.

4. Chew Slowly and savour each bite:

- Eating slowly allows your body to recognize satiety signals, preventing overconsumption. Savouring each bite enhances the pleasure of the meal.

5. Limit Distractions:

- Minimise distractions during meals, such as TV or electronic devices. Creating a peaceful dining environment encourages mindful eating and promotes better digestion.

6. Plan Balanced Meals:

Thoughtfully plan meals that include a balance of carbohydrates, proteins, and healthy fats. This approach helps regulate blood sugar levels and provides sustained energy.

7. Experiment with New Flavors:

Embrace variety in your diet by exploring new flavours and cuisines. This not only adds excitement to meals but also broadens your nutritional intake.

8. Listen to Hunger Cues:

Listen to your body's hunger and fullness signals. Eating when genuinely hungry and stopping when satisfied promotes intuitive eating.

9. Cooking Rituals:
Establishing rituals around cooking, such as setting a pleasant ambiance, can turn meal preparation into a mindful and enjoyable activity.

10. Mindful Grocery Shopping:
- Take the time to read labels and make informed choices when grocery shopping. This mindful approach extends the benefits of healthy eating beyond the kitchen.

11. Gratitude Practice:
- Develop an attitude of thankfulness for the sustenance offered by your meals.
Reflecting on the journey from ingredients to the final dish enhances appreciation.

12. Hydration Awareness:
- Stay mindful of your fluid intake. Water is an essential part of mindful eating and contributes to overall well-being.

By incorporating these tips into your daily routine, you can transform cooking and eating into mindful practices that not only support diabetes management but also enrich your overall quality of life. Mindful choices contribute to a positive relationship with food, fostering a holistic approach to well-being.

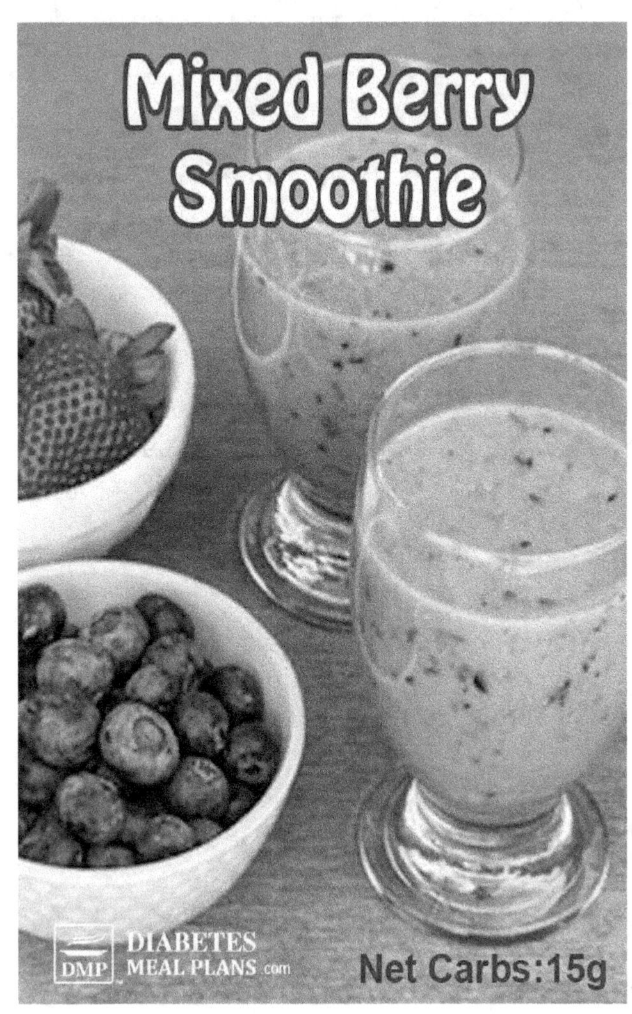

Mixed Berry
Smoothie
DIABETES
DMP MEAL PLANS .com
Net Carbs:15g

CHAPTER TWO

Breakfast Delight

Energising Morning Smoothies

Start your day off right with energising morning smoothies that are both delicious and diabetes-friendly! In The Complete Diabetes Cookbook by the American Diabetes Association (ADA), there are a variety of smoothie recipes that are packed with nutrients and will help you manage your blood sugar levels.

Here are a few of our favourite smoothie recipes from The Complete Diabetes Cookbook:

Berry Blast Smoothie:

Ingredients:
- 1 cup unsweetened almond milk
- 1/2 cup plain Greek yoghourt
- 1/2 cup mixed berries (fresh or frozen)
- 1/2 banana
- 1/2 tsp vanilla extract
- 1/2 cup ice

Instructions:
1. Combine all ingredients in a blender.
2. Blend until smooth.

3. Pour into a glass and enjoy!

This smoothie contains a good balance of carbohydrates, protein, and healthy fats, which will help keep your blood sugar levels stable. The berries provide fibre, which slows down the absorption of sugar into your bloodstream.

Green Goddess Smoothie:

Ingredients:
- 1 cup unsweetened almond milk
- 1/2 cup plain Greek yoghourt
- 1 cup baby spinach
- 1/2 avocado
- 1/2 banana
- 1/2 lime, juiced
- 1/2 cup ice

Instructions:
1. Combine all ingredients in a blender.
2. Blend until smooth.
3. Pour into a glass and enjoy!

This smoothie is a great way to sneak in some extra greens and healthy fats in the morning. The avocado and spinach provide fibre and healthy fats, which will help keep you feeling full and satisfied.

Tropical Paradise Smoothie:

Ingredients:
- 1 cup unsweetened coconut milk
- 1/2 cup plain Greek yoghourt
- 1/2 cup frozen pineapple
- 1/2 banana
- 1/2 tsp vanilla extract
- 1/2 cup ice

Instructions:
1. Combine all ingredients in a blender.
2. Blend until smooth.
3. Pour into a glass and enjoy!

This smoothie is a tropical twist on a classic breakfast smoothie. The pineapple provides natural sweetness and vitamin C, while the coconut milk adds healthy fats and a creamy texture.

Remember to always check the nutrition labels on your ingredients and adjust the serving size as needed to fit your specific dietary needs. Enjoy your energising morning smoothies!

Wholesome Oatmeal Variations

Oatmeal is a nutritious and delicious breakfast option that is perfect for people with diabetes. It is a complex carbohydrate that provides sustained energy throughout the day and helps to regulate blood sugar levels. In this article, we will explore some wholesome oatmeal variations that are both delicious and healthy for people with diabetes.

1. Apple Cinnamon Oatmeal:

This classic combination is a favourite for many people with diabetes as it is low in sugar and high in fibre. To prepare, add 1 chopped apple and 1 teaspoon of cinnamon to 1 cup of oatmeal. Cook according to package directions, then enjoy.

2. Banana Walnut Oatmeal:

This variation is rich in healthy fats and fibre. Add 1 mashed banana and 1/4 cup of chopped walnuts to 1 cup of oatmeal. Cook according to package directions, then enjoy.

3. Berry Blast Oatmeal:

This variation is packed with antioxidants and fibre. Add 1/2 cup of mixed berries (such as strawberries, blueberries, and raspberries) to 1 cup of oatmeal before cooking according to package instructions and enjoy the burst of flavour in every bite!

4. Peanut Butter Banana Oatmeal:

This variation is high in protein and healthy fats from peanut butter and bananas which makes it a filling breakfast option for people with diabetes who need sustained energy throughout the day! Add 2 tablespoons of peanut butter and ½ mashed banana to ½ cup of oatmeal before cooking according to package instructions and enjoy!

5. Pumpkin Spice Oatmeal:

This variation is perfect for fall as it is rich in fibre and pumpkin spice flavour! Add ½ cup of pumpkin puree and ½ teaspoon of pumpkin pie spice to ½ cup of oatmeal before cooking according to package instructions and enjoy!

These variations are not only delicious but also provide a variety of nutrients that are beneficial for people with diabetes such as fibre and healthy fats that help to regulate blood sugar levels and avoid blood sugar rises following meals! Incorporating these wholesome oatmeal variations into your breakfast routine will not only provide sustained energy throughout the day but also help to manage blood sugar levels and promote overall health and wellbeing!

Protein-packed Breakfast Options

When it comes to managing diabetes, breakfast is a crucial meal that can set the tone for blood sugar levels throughout the day. Choosing breakfast options that are high in protein can help slow down the absorption of carbohydrates, preventing spikes in blood sugar. In this article, we will explore some protein-packed breakfast options that are delicious and perfect for diabetics.

Greek Yoghourt Parfait

One cup of Greek yoghurt has about 20 grams of protein, making it a great source of protein. To make this breakfast option, start with plain Greek yoghurt, then add fresh berries, chopped nuts, and a sprinkle of granola. This parfait is not only high in protein but also fibre, which helps to keep you full for longer. For added sweetness without spiking blood sugar levels too much use sugar-free syrup or honey. You can also add a tablespoon of chia seeds for extra protein and omega-3 fatty acids.

Egg White Omelette

Egg whites contain few calories and fat, but are high in protein. One big egg white has around four grams of protein. To make an egg white omelette, whisk two to three egg whites with your choice of vegetables, such as spinach, mushrooms, and bell peppers, and cook in a non-stick pan until set. You can also add a slice of low-carb cheese for extra flavour and protein, but be mindful of portion sizes as cheese can be high in fat and calories.

Cottage Cheese and Fruit Bowl

Cottage cheese is a great source of protein, with one cup containing around 25 grams, and it's also low in fat and calories, making it a perfect breakfast option for diabetics who are watching their weight as well as their blood sugar levels. To make this breakfast option, start with a cup of low-fat cottage cheese, then add fresh fruit such as strawberries, blueberries, and peaches, and a sprinkle of cinnamon for added flavor and blood sugar control benefits due to its low glycemic index rating compared to sugar-sweetened fruits like pineapple or mango, which are high in sugar and should be consumed in moderation by diabetics or avoided altogether in some cases depending on individual blood sugar management needs and preferences, as advised by their healthcare provider or nutritionist/dietitian, who can provide personalized meal planning and guidance based on their unique circumstances and goals, such as weight loss, blood sugar control, or overall health and wellness objectives, and can also help to identify and address any potential food allergies or intolerances that may affect their breakfast choices and meal planning strategies, among other factors that can impact their diabetes management and overall health and wellbeing, such as medication and lifestyle habits like exercise, stress management, and sleep hygiene, which should also be taken into account and addressed as part of a holistic and comprehensive diabetes management plan that is tailored to their individual needs and preferences, and is regularly reviewed and adjusted as needed by their healthcare provider or diabetes care team, which may include a diabetes educator, nutritionist/dietitian, and other healthcare professionals who can provide ongoing support, education, and guidance to help them manage their diabetes effectively and achieve their health and wellness goals over time.

Protein Smoothie

Smoothies are a quick and easy breakfast option, and adding protein powder to them can make them more filling and satisfying. When making a protein smoothie, start with a base of unsweetened almond milk or Greek yogurt, then add protein powder, fresh or frozen fruit, and a handful of spinach or kale for added nutrition. You can also add a tablespoon of chia seeds or flaxseeds for extra fiber and omega-3 fatty acids.

Avocado Toast with Egg

Avocado is a good source of healthy fats and fiber, while whole-grain bread provides complex carbohydrates. To make this breakfast option, start with a slice of whole-grain bread, then mash half an avocado and spread it on the bread. Fry an egg and place it on top of the avocado. You can also add a sprinkle of salt, pepper, and red pepper flakes for added flavour.

Incorporating protein-packed breakfast options into your daily routine can help to manage blood sugar levels, prevent spikes, and keep you full for longer. These solutions are not only tasty, but also healthy and simple to prepare. Remember to always consult with your healthcare provider or diabetes care team for personalised meal planning and guidance based on your unique circumstances and goals, and to regularly review and adjust your meal plan as needed to ensure optimal diabetes management and overall health and wellbeing.

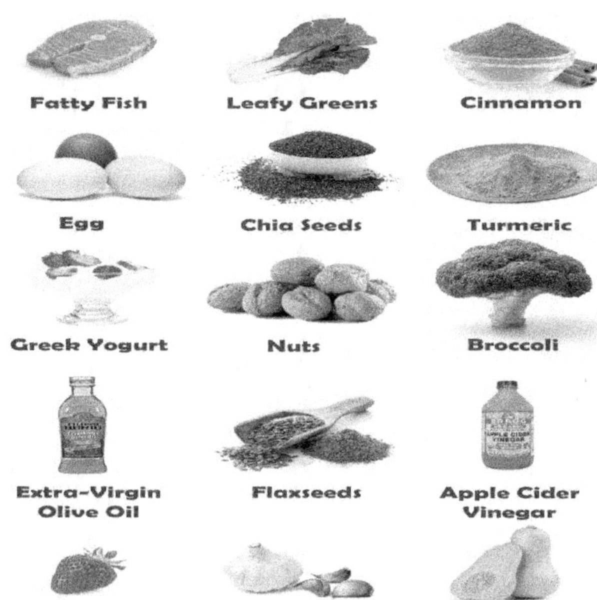

Shirataki Noodles

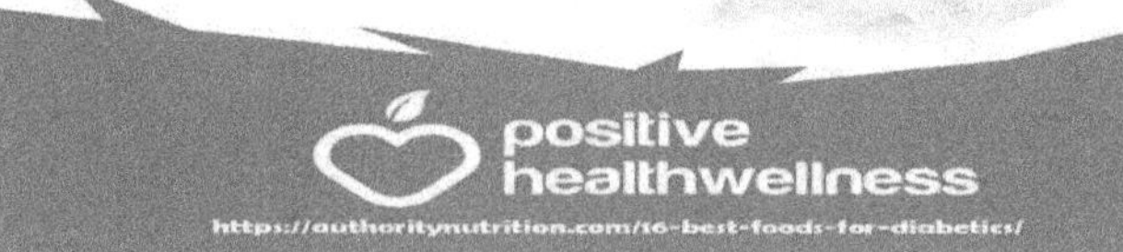

CHAPTER THREE

Lunchtime Favourites

Colourful Salads and Dressings

Salads are a delicious and healthy choice for lunchtime, and adding vibrant colours to them can make them even more appealing. In The Complete Diabetes Cookbook, we have a variety of colourful salad recipes that are not only visually stunning but also packed with nutrients. Here are some of our favourites:

1. Rainbow Quinoa Salad:

This salad is a feast for the eyes, with a rainbow of colours from the red bell pepper, orange carrots, yellow cherry tomatoes, green cucumber, and purple cabbage. Quinoa adds a hearty texture and is a good source of protein for people with diabetes.

2. Mediterranean Chickpea Salad:

This salad is a burst of colours with red cherry tomatoes, yellow bell pepper, green cucumber, and black olives. Chickpeas are a great source of fibre and protein, making this salad a filling and healthy choice.

3. Spicy Tuna Salad:

This salad is a twist on the classic tuna salad, with added spice from jalapeño peppers and red onion. The green lettuce, red tomatoes, and yellow bell pepper make it a colourful and nutritious choice.

4. Grilled Vegetable Salad:

This salad is a medley of colours from the grilled red bell pepper, yellow squash, green zucchini, and orange bell pepper. Grilling adds a smoky flavour and makes the vegetables more tender and delicious.

5. Tropical Fruit Salad:

This salad is a refreshing and colourful mix of tropical fruits, including red watermelon, yellow pineapple, green kiwi, and orange mango. It's a great choice for people with diabetes who want a sweet and healthy treat.

To make these salads even more delicious, we have a variety of dressings that are low in sugar and calories, making them a healthy choice for people with diabetes. Here are some of our favourites:

1. Lemon Vinaigrette:

This dressing is made with fresh lemon juice, olive oil, and Dijon mustard. It's a tangy and refreshing choice that pairs well with most salads.

2. Balsamic Vinaigrette:

This dressing is made with balsamic vinegar, olive oil, and honey. It's a sweet and tangy choice that adds a delicious flavour to salads.

3. Avocado Dressing:

This dressing is made with ripe avocado, lime juice, and Greek yoghourt. It's a creamy and healthy choice that adds a rich flavour to salads.

4. Mustard Vinaigrette:

This dressing is made with Dijon mustard, olive oil, and red wine vinegar. It's a tangy and flavorful choice that adds a zesty kick to salads.

5. Raspberry Vinaigrette:

This dressing is made with fresh raspberries, red wine vinegar, and olive oil. It's a sweet and tart choice that adds a fruity flavour to salads.

In conclusion, colourful salads and dressings are a delicious and healthy choice for lunchtime favourites. The Complete Diabetes Cookbook has a variety of recipes and dressings that are low in sugar and calories, making them a healthy choice for people with diabetes. So, why not try out some of these recipes and dressings today and enjoy a colourful and nutritious lunchtime meal?

Low-Glycemic Sandwich Creations

When it comes to managing diabetes, it's essential to make smart food choices that help regulate blood sugar levels. Sandwiches can be a convenient and satisfying lunch option, but not all fillings are created equal. In The Complete Diabetes Cookbook, we've compiled a list of low-glycemic sandwich creations that are not only delicious but also won't cause a spike in blood sugar.

Grilled Chicken and Avocado Sandwich

Ingredients:
- 2 slices whole-grain bread
- 2 oz grilled chicken breast
- 1/2 avocado, sliced
- 1/4 red onion, sliced
- 1/4 red bell pepper, sliced
- 1 tbsp olive oil
- 1 tbsp balsamic vinegar
- Salt and pepper to taste

Instructions:
1. In a small bowl, whisk together olive oil, balsamic vinegar, salt, and pepper.
2. Toast the bread slices.
3. Layer chicken, avocado, and red onion and bell pepper on one slice of bread.
4. Drizzle the dressing over the filling.
5. Top with the other slice of bread.

Nutritional Information (per serving):
Calories: 350
Carbohydrates: 30g
Protein: 25g
Fat: 15g
Fibre: 8g
Glycemic Index: 35

Tuna Salad Lettuce Wraps

Ingredients:
- 1 can tuna in water, drained
- 1/4 red onion, finely chopped
- 1/4 celery, finely chopped
- 1 tbsp mayonnaise
- 1 tbsp Dijon mustard
- 1 tbsp lemon juice
- Salt and pepper to taste
- 4 large lettuce leaves

Instructions:
1. In a medium bowl, combine tuna, red onion, celery, mayonnaise, Dijon mustard, lemon juice, salt, and pepper.
2. Spoon the tuna salad onto the lettuce leaves.

Nutritional Information (per serving):
Calories: 120
Carbohydrates: 5g
Protein: 18g

Fat: 5g
Fibre: 2g
Glycemic Index: 15

Egg Salad with Spinach

Egg Salad with Spinach

Ingredients:
- 2 hard-boiled eggs, chopped
- 1/4 red onion, finely chopped
- 1/4 celery, finely chopped
- 1 tbsp mayonnaise
- 1 tbsp Dijon mustard
- 1 tbsp lemon juice
- Salt and pepper to taste
- 2 cups baby spinach

Instructions:
1. In a medium bowl, combine eggs, red onion, celery, mayonnaise, Dijon mustard, lemon juice, salt, and pepper.
2. Spread the spinach leaves on a plate.
3. Spoon the egg salad onto the spinach.

Nutritional Information (per serving):
Calories: 150
Carbohydrates: 5g
Protein: 12g
Fat: 10g
Fibre: 2g
Glycemic Index: 15

Ingredients:
- 2 slices whole-grain bread
- 2 oz turkey breast
- 2 tbsp hummus
- 1/4 cucumber, sliced
- 1/4 red bell pepper, sliced
- 1/4 red onion, sliced
- Salt and pepper to taste

Instructions:
1. Spread hummus on one side of each bread slice.
2. Layer turkey, cucumber, bell pepper, and red onion on one slice of bread.
3. Season with salt and pepper.
4. Top with the remaining slice of bread.

Nutritional Information (per serving):
Calories: 320
Carbohydrates: 30g
Protein: 25g
Fat: 12g
Fibre: 6g
Glycemic Index: 35

Grilled Portobello Mushroom and Spinach Sandwich

Ingredients:
- 2 large portobello mushroom caps

- 1 tbsp olive oil
- Salt and pepper to taste
- 2 slices whole-grain bread
- 2 cups baby spinach
- 1/4 red onion, sliced
- 1/4 red bell pepper, sliced

Instructions:
1. Preheat the grill to medium-high heat.
2. Brush mushroom caps with olive oil and season with salt and pepper.
3. Grill mushrooms for 3-4 minutes per side, or until tender.
4. Toast the bread slices.
5. Layer spinach, mushrooms, and red onion and bell pepper on one slice of bread.
6. Top with the remaining slice of bread.

Nutritional Information (per serving):
Calories: 250
Carbohydrates: 25g
Protein: 10g
Fat: 12g
Fibre: 6g
Glycemic Index: 35

These low-glycemic sandwich creations are not only delicious but also packed with nutrients that will help keep blood sugar levels in check. Enjoy!

Hearty Soups for Sustained Energy

Hearty soups are not only delicious but also a great option for sustained energy during lunchtime. They are packed with nutrients, fibre, and protein, which help keep you full and satisfied for longer periods. In The Complete Diabetes Cookbook, we have compiled a list of lunchtime favourites that are not only hearty but also diabetic-friendly.

1. Chicken and Vegetable Soup:

This classic soup is a great choice for sustained energy. It is loaded with protein from the chicken, fibre from the vegetables, and complex carbohydrates from the whole-grain noodles. To make it more filling, add some quinoa or brown rice.

2. Minestrone Soup:

This Italian soup is a nutritional powerhouse. It is loaded with vegetables like spinach, kale, and carrots, which are rich in fibre and vitamins. The addition of white beans and whole-grain pasta makes it a complete meal.

3. Lentil Soup:

Lentils are a great source of protein and fibre, making them an excellent choice for sustained energy. This soup is also rich in iron and other essential minerals. To make it more filling, add some chopped kale or spinach.

4. Butternut Squash Soup:

This soup is rich in fibre and complex carbohydrates, which provide sustained energy. The addition of cinnamon and nutmeg gives it a warm and cosy flavour. To make it more filling, add some cooked quinoa or brown rice.

5. Vegetable and Chickpea Soup:

This soup is loaded with fibre and protein from the vegetables and chickpeas. It's also high in vitamins and minerals. To make it more filling, add some cooked barley or brown rice.

These soups are not only hearty but also diabetic-friendly. They are low in sugar, salt, and saturated fat, making them a healthy choice for lunchtime. They are also easy to prepare and can be made in large batches, making them a convenient option for busy weekdays.

In conclusion, hearty soups are a great choice for sustained energy during lunchtime. They are packed with nutrients, fibre, and protein, which help keep you full and satisfied for longer periods. In The Complete Diabetes Cookbook, we have compiled a list of lunchtime favourites that are not only hearty but also diabetic-friendly. So, next time you're looking for a healthy and filling lunch option, try one of these soups!

CHAPTER FOUR

Dinner Creations

Lean Protein Dishes

In The Complete Diabetes Cookbook, lean protein dishes are a staple for dinner creations. These dishes are not only healthy for individuals with diabetes, but also for anyone looking to maintain a balanced and nutritious diet. Lean protein sources such as chicken, fish, and tofu are low in fat and calories, making them an excellent choice for those watching their weight or managing their blood sugar levels.

Here are a few lean protein dishes from The Complete Diabetes Cookbook that are both delicious and easy to prepare:

Grilled Chicken with Avocado Salsa:

Marinate boneless, skinless chicken breasts in a mixture of lime juice, olive oil, garlic, and cumin. Grill the chicken until cooked through, then serve with a side of avocado salsa made with diced avocado, red onion, cherry tomatoes, lime juice, and cilantro.

Baked Salmon with Lemon and Dill:

Preheat the oven to 400°F. Arrange the salmon fillets on a baking pan lined with parchment paper. Squeeze fresh lemon juice over the fish, then sprinkle with dried dill and a little salt and pepper. Bake for 12 to 15 minutes, or until the salmon is cooked through.

Tofu Stir-Fry:

Cut firm tofu into cubes and stir-fry in a little oil with sliced bell peppers, broccoli, and snow peas. Add garlic, ginger, and soy sauce for flavour, then serve over brown rice.

Grilled Shrimp Skewers:

Thread large shrimp on skewers, alternating with cherry tomatoes and bell pepper strips. Brush the skewers with a mixture of olive oil, lemon juice, and garlic, then grill until the shrimp are pink and cooked through.

Turkey Burgers with Avocado:

Mix ground turkey with diced avocado, chopped cilantro, and a little salt and pepper. Form into patties and grill until fully done. Serve on a whole wheat bun with lettuce, tomato, and a little mustard.

These dishes are not only healthy and delicious, but also easy to prepare, making them perfect for busy weeknights. By incorporating lean protein sources into your dinner creations, you can ensure that you are getting the nutrients you need while managing your blood sugar levels.

Flavorful Vegetarian Entrees

The Complete Diabetes Cookbook offers a wide variety of delicious and healthy vegetarian entrees that are both Flavourful and satisfying. Here are a few options that are perfect for dinner creations:

1. Spicy Black Bean Enchiladas:

These enchiladas are packed with protein and fibre from the black beans, and the spicy sauce adds a delicious kick. To make them, simply mix canned black beans with salsa, cumin, and chilli powder, then roll them up in whole wheat tortillas and bake in the oven.

2. Mushroom Stroganoff:

This vegetarian twist on a classic dish is just as rich and flavorful as the original. Sauté mushrooms, onions, and garlic in a pan, then add vegetable broth, sour cream, and mustard for a creamy sauce. Serve over whole wheat noodles for a hearty and healthy meal.

3. Quinoa Stuffed Peppers:

These stuffed peppers are a great way to incorporate more vegetables and whole grains into your diet. Cook quinoa according to package instructions, then mix with black beans, corn, and salsa. Stuff the mixture into halved bell peppers, then bake until cooked.

4. Lentil Shepherd's Pie:

This vegetarian version of a classic comfort food is just as hearty and satisfying. Cook lentils with vegetable broth, onions, carrots, and celery, then top with mashed sweet potatoes for a delicious and healthy twist.

5. Spinach and Feta Stuffed Portobello Mushrooms:

These stuffed mushrooms are a great way to incorporate more vegetables and protein into your diet. Simply mix spinach, feta cheese, and garlic, then stuff the mixture into portobello mushroom caps and bake in the oven.

These vegetarian entrees are not only flavorful and satisfying, but they are also packed with nutrients and low in sugar, making them a great choice for people with diabetes. With a little creativity, you can create delicious and healthy vegetarian meals that will leave you feeling satisfied and energised.

Smart Carbohydrate Choices

When it comes to managing diabetes, making smart carbohydrate choices is crucial for maintaining stable blood sugar levels.

This is especially true during dinner time as meals consumed later in the day can have a significant impact on overnight blood sugar levels.

In The Complete Diabetes Cookbook, we've compiled a list of smart carbohydrate choices that can be incorporated into delicious dinner creations to help manage diabetes:

- Non-starchy vegetables: These low-carb vegetables such as broccoli, cauliflower, spinach, and Brussels sprouts are packed with fibre and nutrients and can be used as a base for many dinner dishes.

- Whole grains: Choosing whole grains such as brown rice, quinoa, and whole wheat pasta instead of refined grains can provide more fibre and nutrients, helping to slow down carbohydrate absorption and prevent blood sugar spikes.

- Leafy greens: Leafy greens such as lettuce, kale, and collard greens are low in carbohydrates and high in fibre, making them an excellent choice for salads or as a side dish.

- Fruits: Berries such as strawberries, raspberries, and blueberries are low in carbohydrates and high in fibre, making them a great choice for dessert or as a topping for oatmeal or yoghourt for breakfast or dinner creations like fruit salads or grilled fruit skewers for dessert options that won't spike blood sugar levels too much after dinner time consumption!

- Legumes: Legumes such as lentils, chickpeas, and black beans are high in fibre and protein, helping to slow down carbohydrate absorption and prevent blood sugar spikes. Incorporating these smart carbohydrate choices into dinner creations can help manage diabetes by providing a balance of nutrients, fibre, and protein to promote stable blood sugar levels.

Here are some dinner ideas that incorporate these smart carbohydrate choices:

1. Grilled Chicken and Vegetable Skewers: Thread chicken breast, bell peppers, zucchini, and mushrooms onto skewers and grill until cooked through. Serve with a serving of brown rice and steamed broccoli.

2. Quinoa and Black Bean Salad: Cook quinoa according to package instructions and mix with black beans, cherry tomatoes, avocado, and a lime vinaigrette. Serve with a side of grilled asparagus.

3. Spinach and Feta Stuffed Chicken Breast: Pound chicken breasts thin and stuffed with

spinach and feta cheese. Bake in the oven
until cooked through and serve with a side
of roasted Brussels sprouts.

4. Grilled Salmon and Asparagus: Grill salmon
    and serve with steamed asparagus and a
    side of brown rice.

5. Lentil and Vegetable Stir-Fry: Sauté lentils,
    bell peppers, onions, and broccoli in a pan
    with garlic and ginger. Serve with a serving
    of cooked brown rice. These dinner ideas
    provide a balance of smart carbohydrate
    choices, protein, and healthy fats to
    promote stable blood sugar levels and help
    manage diabetes.

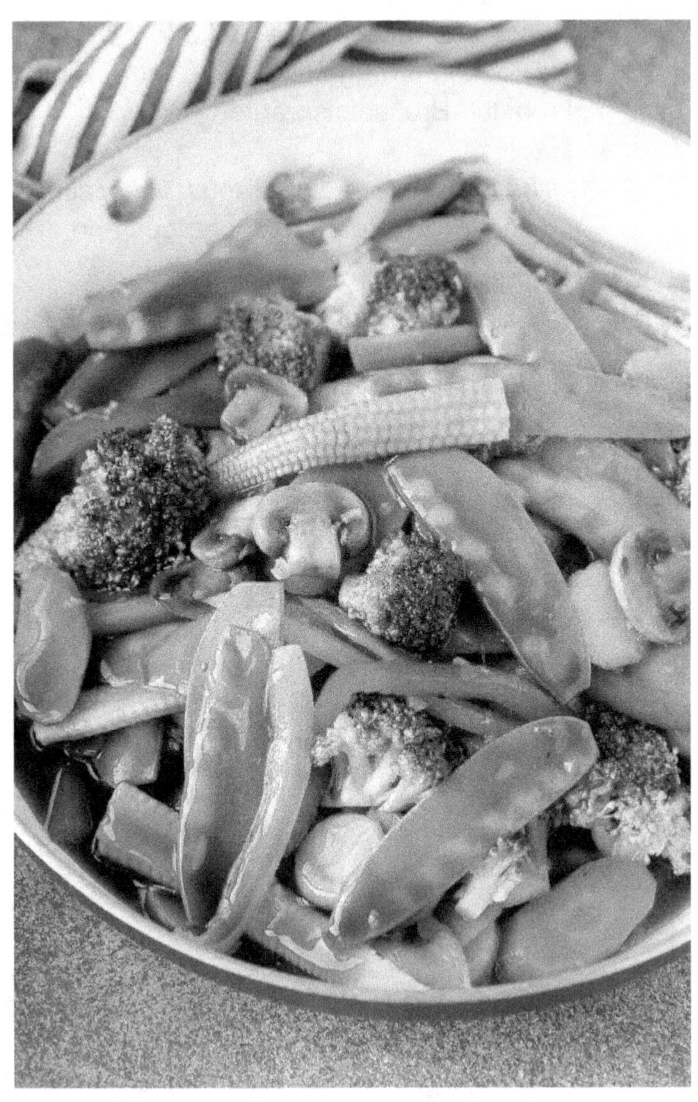

CHAPTER FIVE

Snacks and Appetisers

Nutrient-Rich Snack Ideas

In The Complete Diabetes Cookbook, there are numerous snack and appetisers ideas that are not only delicious but also packed with essential nutrients. Here are some nutrient-rich snack ideas that are perfect for managing diabetes:

- Roasted Chickpeas: Chickpeas are a great source of protein and fibre, making them an excellent choice for managing blood sugar levels. Roast them with some spices like cumin, paprika, and garlic powder for a crunchy and flavorful snack.

- Apple Slices with Almond Butter: Apples are rich in fibre, which helps slow down the absorption of sugar into the bloodstream. Pair them with a tablespoon of almond butter, which is high in healthy fats and protein, for a satisfying and nutritious snack.

- Carrot and Celery Sticks with Hummus: Carrots and celery are low in calories and high in fibre, making them an ideal snack for managing diabetes. Dip them in hummus, which is rich in protein and healthy fats, for a nutrient-dense snack.

- Greek Yoghourt with Berries: Greek yoghourt is high in protein, which helps keep blood sugar levels stable. Add some fresh berries, which are low in sugar and high in fibre, for a sweet and satisfying snack.

- Edamame: Edamame is a soybean that is rich in protein and fibre. Boil them and sprinkle some sea salt for a healthy and delicious snack.

- Baked Sweet Potato Chips: Sweet potatoes are rich in fibre and vitamins, making them a nutritious choice for managing diabetes. Bake them into thin chips for a crunchy and flavourful snack.

- Hard-Boiled Eggs: Eggs are an excellent source of protein, which helps keep blood sugar levels stable. Hard-boil them for a quick and convenient snack.

- Cucumber and Tomato Salad: Cucumbers and tomatoes are low in calories and high in fibre and water content, making them an ideal snack for managing diabetes. Toss them together with some olive oil and vinegar for a refreshing and nutritious salad.

- Turkey Roll-Ups: Roll up some turkey slices with some avocado, lettuce, and tomato for a protein-packed and low-carb snack.

- Roasted Nuts: Nuts are rich in healthy fats, protein, and fibre. Roast them with some spices like cinnamon and nutmeg for a sweet and nutritious snack.

Incorporating these nutrient-rich snack ideas into your diet can help manage diabetes and promote overall health. Remember to always consult with a healthcare professional for personalised dietary advice.

Guilt-Free Appetisers for Any Occasion

As someone with diabetes, it can be challenging to find appetiser options that are both delicious and guilt-free. However, with a little creativity and some healthy ingredient swaps, you can whip up a variety of appetisers that are perfect for any occasion. Here are some ideas to get you started:

Baked Sweet Potato Chips

Sweet potatoes are a great alternative to regular potatoes because they are lower on the glycemic index, meaning they won't cause a spike in blood sugar levels like regular potatoes can do for people with diabetes or anyone looking for healthier options for snacks and appetisers alike! Slice sweet potatoes thinly and toss them with olive oil and your favourite seasonings (such as garlic powder and paprika). Bake them at 400°F for 15-20 minutes or until crispy.

Grilled Vegetable Skewers

Vegetables are a great source of fibre and nutrients, making them an excellent choice for people with diabetes. Thread your favourite veggies (such as bell peppers, mushrooms, and zucchini) onto skewers and grill them until tender. Drizzle them with a little olive oil and lemon juice for added flavour.

Caprese Skewers

Caprese skewers are a classic appetiser that's both delicious and healthy. Thread cherry tomatoes, mozzarella balls, and basil leaves onto skewers. Drizzle them with balsamic vinegar and olive oil for a simple and tasty appetisers.

Avocado Deviled Eggs

Deviled eggs are a classic appetiser, but you can make them a little healthier by swapping out some of the mayo for mashed avocado. Mash the yolks with avocado, lime juice, and your favourite seasonings (such as cumin and chilli powder).

Spoon the mixture back into the egg whites and sprinkle with paprika.

Spicy Roasted Chickpeas

Chickpeas are a great source of protein and fibre, making them an excellent choice for people with diabetes. Toss canned chickpeas with olive oil, cumin, chilli powder, and a little cayenne pepper. Roast them in the oven at 400°F for 20-25 minutes or until crispy.

Cucumber and Cream Cheese Roll-Ups

Cucumber roll-ups are a refreshing and healthy appetisers option. Spread a little cream cheese onto a cucumber slice and roll it up. Garnish with a sprinkle of dill or chives.

Mini Turkey Burgers

Turkey burgers are a leaner alternative to traditional beef burgers, making them a great choice for people with diabetes. Cook mini turkey burgers and serve them on whole-grain buns with lettuce, tomato, and avocado.

Zucchini Fritters

Zucchini fritters are a delicious and healthy appetiser option. Grate zucchini and squeeze out the excess moisture. Mix the zucchini with eggs, almond flour, and your favourite seasonings (such as garlic powder and parsley). Fry them in a little olive oil until crispy.

Baked Apple Chips

Apples are a great source of fibre and nutrients, making them an excellent choice for people with diabetes. Slice apples thinly and toss them with cinnamon and a little honey. Bake them at 200°F for 2-3 hours or until crispy.

Mini Bell Pepper Nachos

Nachos are a classic appetiser, but you can make them a little healthier by swapping out the tortilla chips for bell pepper slices. Top the bell pepper slices with black beans, salsa, and a little shredded cheese. Broil them in the oven until the cheese melts and bubbles.

These guilt-free appetisers are not only healthy but also delicious and easy to prepare. They're perfect for any occasion, whether you're hosting a party or just looking for a healthy snack option. Enjoy!

CHAPTER SIX

Desserts with a Twist

Sugar-Free Sweet Endings

In The Complete Diabetes Cookbook, sugar-free sweet endings for desserts with a twist are a staple for those with diabetes who still crave something sweet after meals. These recipes are not only sugar-free but also incorporate unique flavours and ingredients to make them stand out from traditional desserts.

One such recipe is the Chocolate Avocado Mousse. This mousse is made with ripe avocados, unsweetened cocoa powder, almond milk, and a touch of vanilla extract. The avocados provide a creamy texture, while the cocoa powder adds rich chocolate flavour. This mousse is not only sugar-free but also packed with healthy fats and fibre.

Another recipe that's a crowd-pleaser is the Berry Sorbet. This sorbet is made with a mix of fresh berries, lemon juice, and water. The berries are blended until smooth, and then the mixture is frozen until it reaches a sorbet-like consistency. This sorbet is not only sugar-free but also low in calories and high in fibre.

For those who prefer a more indulgent dessert, the Cinnamon Apple Crisp is a great option. This crisp is made with sliced apples, cinnamon, and a crumbly oat and almond flour topping. The apples are cooked until they are soft and caramelised, while the topping adds a crunchy texture. This crisp is not only sugar-free but also gluten-free and low in carbohydrates.

Finally, the Coconut Chia Seed Pudding is a unique twist on traditional pudding. This pudding is made with chia seeds, coconut milk, and a touch of vanilla extract. The chia seeds absorb moisture, resulting in a pudding-like consistency. This pudding is not only sugar-free but also high in fibre and healthy fats.

In conclusion, The Complete Diabetes Cookbook offers a variety of sugar-free sweet endings for desserts with a twist. These recipes are not only delicious but also healthy and nutritious, making them a great option for those with diabetes who still want to indulge in something sweet. With these recipes, you can satisfy your sweet tooth without compromising your health.

Fruitful and Satisfying Treats

In The Complete Diabetes Cookbook, author and nutritionist Cheryl Forberg offers a collection of dessert recipes that are both fruitful and satisfying, with a twist that sets them apart from traditional sugary treats. These desserts are not only delicious but also diabetes-friendly, as they are low in sugar and high in fibre, healthy fats, and protein.

One such recipe is the Grilled Pineapple with Cinnamon and Coconut. This dessert is a refreshing twist on traditional grilled fruit, as the sweetness of the pineapple is enhanced by the smoky flavour of the grill and the warm spice of cinnamon. The addition of unsweetened coconut adds a tropical flair and a healthy dose of healthy fats.

Another standout recipe is the Chocolate Avocado Pudding. This rich and decadent dessert is made with ripe avocados, unsweetened cocoa powder, and a touch of vanilla extract. The avocados provide healthy fats and creaminess, while the cocoa powder adds a deep chocolate flavour without the need for added sugar. This pudding is also high in fibre, thanks to the addition of chia seeds, which help to keep you feeling full and satisfied.

For those with a sweet tooth, the Berry Balsamic Tart is a must-try. This tart combines fresh berries with a tangy balsamic glaze, which adds a unique and unexpected flavour to the dessert. The crust is made with almond flour and coconut oil, which provides a healthy dose of healthy fats and protein. This tart is also low in sugar, as the sweetness comes from the berries and a touch of honey.

In addition to these recipes, The Complete Diabetes Cookbook also includes a variety of other fruitful and satisfying desserts, such as Apple Cinnamon Oatmeal, Banana Almond Butter Bites, and Mixed Berry Sorbet. These recipes are not only delicious but also easy to prepare, making them the perfect addition to any diabetes-friendly diet.

In conclusion, The Complete Diabetes Cookbook offers a collection of fruitful and satisfying desserts with a twist that are both diabetes-friendly and delicious. These recipes are low in sugar, high in fibre, and packed with healthy fats and protein, making them a guilt-free indulgence. Whether you're looking for a refreshing fruit salad, a rich chocolate pudding, or a tart berry dessert, this cookbook has something for everyone.

Mindful Portion Control

In The Complete Diabetes Cookbook, mindful portion control for desserts is taken to the next level with a creative twist. The cookbook recognizes that indulging in sweet treats is a part of life, but it's essential to do so in moderation, especially for individuals with diabetes. The cookbook offers a variety of dessert recipes that are not only delicious but also portion-controlled, making it easier to enjoy without overindulging.

One of the unique features of this cookbook is the emphasis on mindfulness. It encourages readers to savour every bite, appreciate the flavours and textures, and avoid mindless snacking. This approach helps individuals make more conscious choices about their dessert intake and prevents overeating.

The cookbook also offers a twist by incorporating healthy ingredients into desserts. For instance, the recipe for Chocolate Avocado Pudding uses avocado as a base, which is rich in healthy fats and fibre. The recipe for Berry Chia Seed Pudding uses chia seeds, which are high in protein and fibre, making it a more filling and nutritious dessert option.

Another twist is the use of natural sweeteners like honey, maple syrup, and stevia instead of refined sugar. These sweeteners not only add flavour but also provide additional nutrients like antioxidants and minerals.

The cookbook also offers tips for portion control, such as using smaller plates, measuring ingredients, and dividing desserts into individual servings. These strategies help individuals stay mindful of their dessert intake and prevent overeating.

In conclusion, The Complete Diabetes Cookbook offers a unique approach to mindful portion control for desserts with a twist. The cookbook's emphasis on mindfulness, use of healthy ingredients, and natural sweeteners makes it an excellent resource for individuals with diabetes who want to enjoy desserts without compromising their health. By following the cookbook's tips and recipes, individuals can indulge in sweet treats in moderation and savour every bite.

CHAPTER SEVEN

Kitchen Tips and Tricks

Ingredient Substitutions for Healthier Cooking

Ingredient substitutions can be a game changer when it comes to making healthier choices while cooking delicious meals that won't compromise flavour or texture too much! Here are some tips for ingredient substitutions that can help you make your cooking more diabetes-friendly:

Sugar Substitutions:

Instead of using white sugar or brown sugar that are high on calories with little nutritional value, try using natural sweeteners like honey or pure maple syrup that are rich in antioxidants and minerals. Stevia, a plant-based, zero-calorie sweetener, is another great option that is much sweeter than sugar, so you'll need less of it.

Fat Substitutions:

To reduce the amount of saturated and trans fats in your cooking, replace butter, shortening, and lard with healthier fats like olive oil, avocado oil, or canola oil. These fats are rich in monounsaturated and polyunsaturated fats, which can help lower cholesterol levels and reduce the risk of heart disease.

Flour Substitutions:

Whole wheat flour is a healthier alternative to white flour because it contains more fibre and nutrients like B vitamins and iron. You can also try using almond flour or coconut flour instead of wheat flour for a gluten-free option that is lower in carbohydrates and higher in protein and healthy fats.

Dairy Substitutions:

For those who are lactose intolerant or prefer non-dairy options, you can replace regular milk with almond milk, soy milk, or coconut milk in your recipes without compromising taste or texture too much. Greek yoghourt is also a great option because it is high in protein and low in sugar compared to regular yoghourt.

Spice Substitutions:

Instead of using salt to add flavour to your dishes, try using herbs and spices like garlic, ginger, cumin, or turmeric that can add depth of flavour without adding extra calories or sodium. These spices also have health benefits like anti-inflammatory properties that can help reduce the risk of chronic diseases like diabetes and heart disease.

By making these ingredient substitutions, you can create healthier and more diabetes-friendly meals that are still delicious and satisfying! Remember to always consult with a healthcare professional or a registered dietitian for personalised nutrition advice based on your specific needs and preferences.

Smart Cooking Techniques for Diabetes-Friendly Meals

Smart cooking techniques are essential for preparing diabetes-friendly meals that are not only healthy but also delicious.

Here are some kitchen tips and tricks for smart cooking techniques that you can find in The Complete Diabetes Cookbook:

1. **<u>Grilling:</u>** Grilling is a great way to cook diabetes-friendly meals because it helps to retain the natural flavours and nutrients of the food. Grilling also helps to reduce the amount of fat and calories in the food. Some tips for grilling diabetes-friendly meals include:

- Choose lean cuts of meat, such as chicken breasts, turkey burgers, and fish.

- Marinate the meat in a low-sugar marinade to add flavour without adding extra calories.

- Use a grill basket to cook vegetables, such as bell peppers, onions, and zucchini, without adding extra oil.

2. **<u>Steaming</u>:** Steaming is a healthy cooking technique that helps to retain the nutrients and flavours of the food. Steaming also helps to reduce the amount of fat and calories in the food. Some tips for steaming diabetes-friendly meals include:

- Use a steamer basket to steam vegetables, such as broccoli, carrots, and green beans.

- Add a little bit of flavour to the vegetables by steaming them with garlic, ginger, or lemon juice.

- Use a rice cooker to steam rice without adding extra oil.

3. **<u>Roasting</u>:** Roasting is a delicious way to cook diabetes-friendly meals because it helps to bring out the natural flavours of the food. Roasting also helps to reduce the amount of fat and calories in the food. Some tips for roasting diabetes-friendly meals include:

- Use a roasting pan to roast vegetables, such as sweet potatoes, Brussels sprouts, and cauliflower.

- Add a little bit of olive oil and seasoning to the vegetables before roasting.

- Use a meat thermometer to make sure the meat is cooked to the correct temperature.

4. Sautéing: Sautéing is a quick and easy way to cook diabetes-friendly meals because it helps to retain the natural flavours and nutrients of the food. Sautéing also helps to reduce the amount of fat and calories in the food. Some tips for sautéing diabetes-friendly meals include:

- Use a non-stick pan to sauté vegetables, such as mushrooms, spinach, and bell peppers.

- Add a little bit of olive oil and seasoning to the vegetables before sautéing.

- Use a lid to cover the pan and steam the vegetables for a few minutes.

5. Baking: Baking is a healthy cooking technique that helps to retain the nutrients and flavours of the food. Baking also helps to reduce the amount of fat and calories in the food. Some tips for baking diabetes-friendly meals include:

- Use a baking dish to bake vegetables, such as asparagus, tomatoes, and eggplant.

- Add a little bit of olive oil and seasoning to the vegetables before baking.

- Use a meat thermometer to make sure the meat is cooked to the correct temperature.

By using these smart cooking techniques, you can prepare diabetes-friendly meals that are not only healthy but also delicious. The Complete Diabetes Cookbook provides many more tips and tricks for preparing diabetes-friendly meals, as well as a wide variety of delicious recipes.

Efficient Meal Planning and Preparation

Meal planning and preparation can be a daunting task, especially for individuals with diabetes who need to manage their blood sugar levels. However, with a little bit of organisation and some kitchen tips and tricks, mealtime can become less stressful and more enjoyable. Here are some efficient meal planning and preparation ideas for those with diabetes:

- Plan ahead: Set aside some time each week to plan your meals for the upcoming days or weeks ahead. This will help you stay organised and ensure that you have all the necessary ingredients on hand when it comes time to prepare your meals. You can also take advantage of meal planning apps or websites that offer diabetes-friendly recipes and meal plans for convenience.

- Batch cook: Consider preparing larger portions of meals that can be portioned out and stored in the fridge or freezer for later use. This can save time and money in the long run, as you won't have to cook as often. Just be sure to label and date your meals to keep track of what's inside.

- Use a slow cooker: Slow cookers are a great tool for preparing diabetes-friendly meals, as they allow you to cook large batches of food with minimal effort. Simply add your ingredients to the slow cooker in the morning, and by dinner time, you'll have a delicious and healthy meal ready to go.

- Keep it simple: Don't feel like you have to create elaborate meals every night. Sometimes, the simplest dishes can be the most satisfying. Consider preparing stir-fries, grilled chicken and vegetables, or a simple salad with a homemade vinaigrette. These meals are easy to prepare and can be customised to fit your dietary needs.

- Use a food scale: Accurately measuring your portion sizes is crucial for managing your blood sugar levels. Invest in a food scale to help you portion out your meals accurately. This will also help you avoid overeating, which can lead to spikes in blood sugar.

- Experiment with spices and herbs: Adding flavour to your meals can make them more enjoyable and help you avoid adding excess salt or sugar. Consider experimenting with spices and herbs like cumin, coriander, and basil to add flavour to your meals without adding extra calories.

- Don't forget about snacks: Snacks can be a great way to keep your blood sugar levels stable between meals. Consider preparing healthy snacks like apple slices with almond butter, carrot sticks with hummus, or a small handful of nuts. These snacks are easy to prepare and can be taken on the go.

By following these tips and tricks, you can make meal planning and preparation more efficient and enjoyable, while also managing your blood sugar levels. Remember to always consult with your healthcare provider for personalised dietary advice.

CHAPTER EIGHT

Eating Out with Diabetes

Navigating Restaurant Menus

Eating out with diabetes can be a challenge, but with a little bit of planning and knowledge, it's possible to enjoy a delicious meal without compromising your health. Here are some tips for navigating restaurant menus when you have diabetes:

1. Look for healthy options:

Many restaurants now offer healthy options, such as grilled chicken, salads, and vegetable dishes. These options are typically lower in calories, fat, and carbohydrates, making them a great choice for people with diabetes.

2. Be aware of portion sizes:

Restaurant portions are often larger than what you would eat at home. Consider splitting a meal with a friend or taking half of it home for later.

3. Watch out for hidden carbs:

Some dishes, such as pasta dishes and sandwiches, can be surprisingly high in carbohydrates. Be sure to check the menu for the carbohydrate content of each dish.

4. Choose healthy fats:

When selecting a dish, opt for healthy fats, such as olive oil, avocado, and nuts, instead of saturated and trans fats.

5. Limit alcohol:

Alcohol can cause your blood sugar to drop, so it's best to limit your intake. If you do choose to drink, opt for a glass of wine instead of a cocktail, and be sure to eat something beforehand to prevent a drop in blood sugar.

6. Don't be afraid to ask questions:

If you're not sure about the carbohydrate content of a dish, don't be afraid to ask the server or the chef. They may be able to provide you with more information or suggest a lower carb option.

7. Be mindful of sauces and dressings:

Many sauces and dressings are high in carbohydrates and calories. Consider asking for dressing on the side or opting for a vinaigrette instead of a creamy dressing.

8. Don't forget about dessert:

If you have a sweet tooth, consider sharing a dessert with a friend or opting for a fruit-based dessert, such as fruit sorbet or fresh fruit.

Remember, the most important thing is to enjoy your meal and not feel deprived. With a little bit of planning and knowledge, you can enjoy a delicious meal without compromising your health.

Making Healthy Choices at Cafes and Fast Food Outlets

Eating out at cafes and fast food outlets can be challenging for people with diabetes, as many menu items are high in sugar, salt, and unhealthy fats. However, with a little bit of planning and knowledge, it's possible to make healthy choices that won't derail your diabetes management plan. Here are some tips for making smart choices at cafes and fast food outlets:

Check the menu online before you go:

Many cafes and fast food chains have their menus available online, which can help you make informed decisions before you even step inside. Look for items that are labelled as "healthy" or "low-carb" and read the nutrition information to make sure they fit into your meal plan goals for carbohydrates (carbs), fat intake (fats), calories (calories), sodium (salt), fibre (fibre), protein (protein), etc.. This can save time during your visit as well!

Choose whole foods:

When possible opt for whole foods such as grilled chicken or fish instead of fried items or processed foods such as burgers or sandwiches. These options tend to be lower in calories, fat, and sodium, and higher in protein and fibre.

Many sauces and dressings are high in sugar, salt, and unhealthy fats. Ask for dressings and sauces on the side, and use them sparingly. Alternatively, you can ask for a vinaigrette dressing instead of a creamy dressing, which is usually lower in calories and fat.

Limit your intake of carbohydrates:

Carbohydrates can cause blood sugar spikes, so it's essential to monitor your intake. Choose menu items that are lower in carbs, such as a grilled chicken salad with vinaigrette dressing, or a veggie wrap with whole-grain bread.

Be mindful of portion sizes:

Fast food portions are often much larger than what you need. Consider splitting a meal with a friend or taking half of it home for later.

Don't forget about hydration:

Drink plenty of water throughout your meal, and limit your intake of sugary drinks such as soda or juice.

Be aware of hidden sugars:

Many menu items, such as smoothies or fruit-flavoured yoghourt, can be surprisingly high in sugar. Always check the nutrition label or ask the server for the sugar content.

If you have a sweet tooth, consider choosing a fruit-based dessert, such as fresh fruit or a fruit salad, instead of a sugary dessert. By following these tips, you can make healthy choices at cafes and fast food outlets that will support your diabetes management plan.

Remember to always consult with your healthcare provider or a registered dietitian for personalised advice on managing your diabetes through diet.

Strategies for Social Dining

As someone with diabetes, dining out can be a challenging experience. It's not always easy to find healthy and satisfying options that fit into your meal plan. However, with a little bit of planning and strategy, social dining can be enjoyable and manageable. Here are some tips to help you eat out with diabetes:

- ☐ Research the restaurant: Before heading out, take a look at the menu online. This will give you an idea of what options are available and help you make informed choices. Look for dishes that are high in protein, fibre, and healthy fats, and avoid items that are high in sugar, salt, and unhealthy fats.

☐ Communicate with the server: Let your server know that you have diabetes and need some guidance. They can help you make choices that fit your needs and provide information about portion sizes and ingredient substitutions. Don't be afraid to ask questions about the preparation methods and ingredients used in each dish.

☐ Watch your portions: Restaurant portions are often larger than what you need. Consider sharing a meal with a friend or taking half of your dish home for later. You can also ask for a to-go box when your meal arrives and portion it out yourself.

☐ Choose healthier options: Opt for grilled, baked, or broiled dishes instead of fried foods. Choose whole-grain breads and pasta instead of white bread and pasta. And don't forget to include plenty of vegetables and salad greens to help fill you up.

☐ Be mindful of sauces and dressings: Many sauces and dressings are high in sugar, salt, and unhealthy fats. Ask for dressings and sauces on the side, or opt for healthier alternatives like lemon and olive oil.

☐ Watch your alcohol intake: Alcohol can cause your blood sugar to drop, which can be dangerous if you're not prepared. Limit your alcohol intake and pair it with a meal that includes protein and fibre to help slow down the absorption of alcohol into your bloodstream.

- ☐ Don't forget about dessert: It's okay to indulge in a sweet treat once in a while, but choose wisely. Look for options that are lower in sugar and higher in fibre, like fruit or sorbet. And consider sharing a dessert with a friend to help cut down on portion sizes.

By following these strategies, you can enjoy social dining while managing your diabetes. Remember to always prioritise your health and well-being, and don't be afraid to speak up and ask questions. With a little bit of planning and communication, dining out can be a delicious and enjoyable experience.

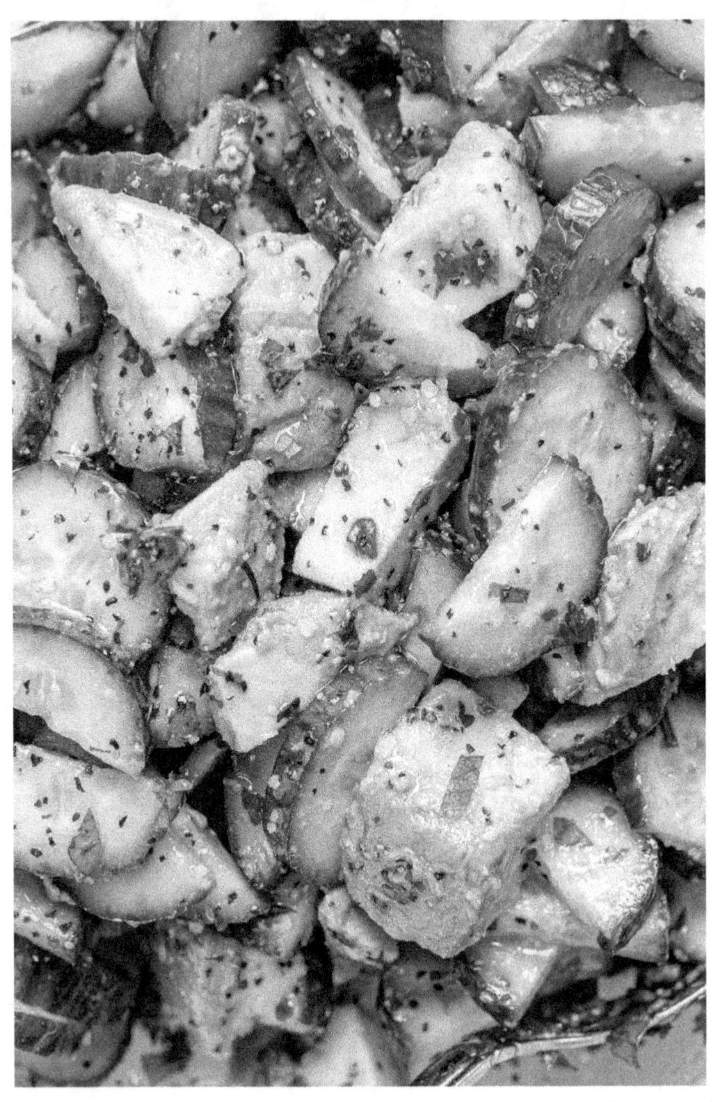

CHAPTER NINE

Success stories

Real-life Experiences of Diabetes Management Through Cooking

The Complete Diabetes Cookbook is a comprehensive resource for individuals living with diabetes who are looking for healthy and delicious meal options that will help them manage their condition effectively through cooking techniques and recipes that are specifically designed for diabetes management purposes. In this article we will explore some real-life experiences of diabetes management through cooking as shared by individuals who have successfully implemented these techniques in their daily lives using recipes from The Complete Diabetes Cookbook as a guide:

1. **Sarah' s Story:** Sarah was diagnosed with type 2 diabetes a few years ago and was struggling to manage her blood sugar levels through medication alone until she discovered The Complete Diabetes Cookbook while browsing online for diabetes management resources. She started incorporating the recipes from the cookbook into her daily diet and noticed a significant improvement in her blood sugar levels within a few weeks. One of her favourite recipes from the cookbook is the Quinoa

Salad with Roasted Vegetables, which is packed with fibre, protein, and healthy fats that help regulate blood sugar levels. Sarah says that she now looks forward to mealtime instead of dreading it because she knows that she has access to delicious and nutritious recipes that will help her manage her diabetes effectively.

2. John' s Story: John was diagnosed with type 1 diabetes at a young age and struggled with managing his blood sugar levels throughout his teenage years. He turned to The Complete Diabetes Cookbook as a resource for healthy meal options that would help him manage his condition more effectively. One of his favourite recipes from the cookbook is the Grilled Chicken with Mango-Avocado Salad, which is low in carbohydrates and high in fibre, protein, and healthy fats. John says that he now enjoys cooking healthy meals for himself and his family using recipes from The Complete Diabetes Cookbook, which has helped him maintain stable blood sugar levels and improve his overall health and wellbeing.

3. Maria' s Story: Maria was diagnosed with gestational diabetes during her pregnancy and was worried about how she would manage her blood sugar levels while still enjoying delicious meals. She turned to The Complete Diabetes Cookbook for healthy and diabetes-friendly recipes that would help her manage her condition during her pregnancy. One of her favourite recipes from the cookbook is the Baked Salmon with Asparagus and Lemon, which is low in carbohydrates and high in omega-3 fatty acids, which are essential for foetal brain development. Maria says that she now enjoys cooking healthy meals for herself and her family using recipes from The Complete Diabetes Cookbook, which has helped her manage her gestational diabetes effectively and maintain a healthy weight throughout her pregnancy. These real-life experiences demonstrate the power of diabetes management through cooking techniques and recipes that are specifically designed for diabetes management purposes. The Complete Diabetes Cookbook provides individuals living with diabetes with a wealth of healthy and delicious meal options that are easy to prepare and incorporate into their daily diet, helping them manage their condition more effectively and improve their overall health and wellbeing.

Overcoming Challenges and Celebrating Victories

The Complete Diabetes Cookbook is more than just a collection of delicious recipes for individuals living with diabetes; it is also a guide for overcoming challenges and celebrating victories on the road to success. The cookbook recognizes that managing diabetes is not an easy feat, and it provides practical tips and inspiring success stories to help individuals navigate the challenges and celebrate their victories.

One of the significant challenges of managing diabetes is maintaining a healthy diet while enjoying delicious meals. The cookbook addresses this challenge by providing a wide variety of recipes that are low in sugar, carbohydrates, and saturated fats. The recipes are also rich in fibre, protein, and healthy fats, which help to keep blood sugar levels stable and promote overall health.

For instance, one success story featured in the cookbook is that of Susan, who was diagnosed with type 2 diabetes. Susan struggled with managing her blood sugar levels and found it challenging to stick to a healthy diet. However, she discovered the cookbook and started incorporating its recipes into her daily meals. She noticed a significant improvement in her blood sugar levels and felt more energised and focused throughout the day. Susan's success story is a testament to the power of healthy eating in managing diabetes.

Another challenge of managing diabetes is staying active and maintaining a healthy weight. The cookbook addresses this challenge by providing tips on how to incorporate physical activity into daily routines and how to make healthy food choices when dining out or travelling. The cookbook also includes recipes that are easy to prepare and can be taken on the go, making it easier for individuals to maintain a healthy diet while travelling.

For instance, one success story featured in the cookbook is that of John, who was overweight and had high blood sugar levels. John started following the cookbook's tips on healthy eating and physical activity, and he lost a significant amount of weight. He also noticed a significant improvement in his blood sugar levels and felt more confident and energetic. John's success story is a testament to the importance of a healthy lifestyle in managing diabetes.

Celebrating victories is also crucial in managing diabetes. The cookbook encourages individuals to celebrate their successes, no matter how small, and to use them as motivation to continue making healthy choices. The cookbook also includes tips on how to make healthy food choices when dining out or travelling, making it easier for individuals to maintain a healthy diet while enjoying life's pleasures.

For instance, one success story featured in the cookbook is that of Sarah, who was hesitant to try new foods and felt overwhelmed by the prospect of managing her diabetes. Sarah started following the cookbook's tips on healthy eating and discovered new foods that she enjoyed. She also started experimenting with new recipes and found that she could enjoy delicious meals while managing her diabetes. Sarah's success story is a testament to the importance of trying new things and celebrating small victories in managing diabetes.

In conclusion, The Complete Diabetes Cookbook is more than just a collection of delicious recipes; it is a guide for overcoming challenges and celebrating victories on the road to success. The cookbook provides practical tips, inspiring success stories, and delicious recipes to help individuals manage their diabetes and enjoy life's pleasures. By following the cookbook's tips and celebrating small victories, individuals can overcome the challenges of managing diabetes and achieve their health goals.

CONCLUSION

The Complete Diabetes Cookbook offers a wealth of delicious and nutritious recipes specifically designed for individuals with diabetes or those looking to maintain a healthy lifestyle. The cookbook provides detailed nutritional information for each recipe, making it easy to manage carbohydrate intake and blood sugar levels. The cookbook also offers tips on meal planning, ingredient substitutions, and cooking techniques to help readers make informed choices about their diet. With a diverse range of recipes from around the world, The Complete Diabetes Cookbook is an essential resource for anyone looking to enjoy delicious meals while managing their diabetes or promoting overall health and wellbeing.

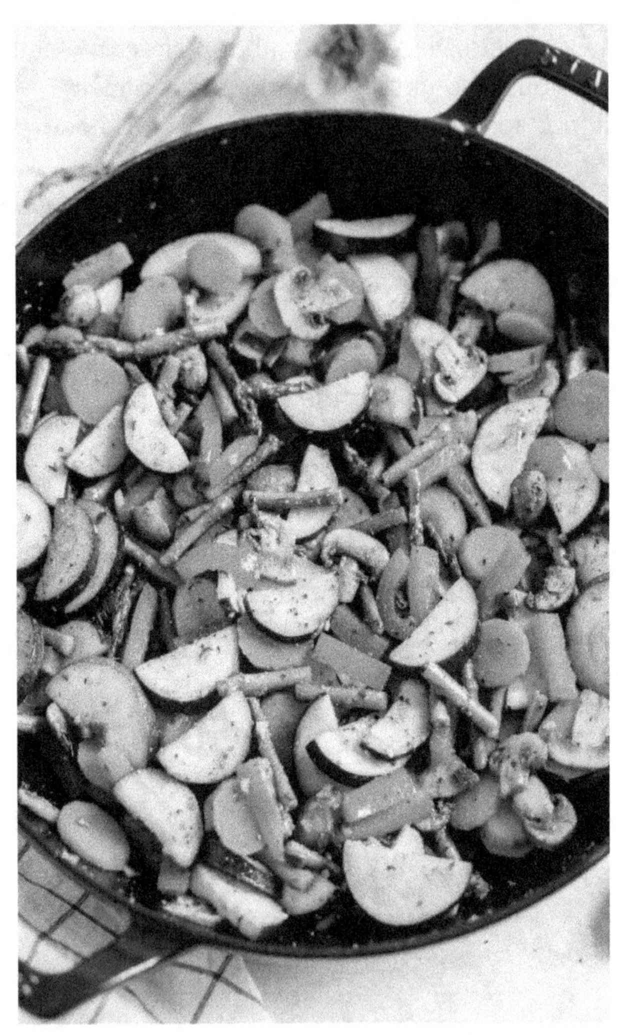